M000198451

Too Pregnant to Move

Copyright © 2019 by Rockridge Press, Emeryville, California

No part of this publication may be reproduced, stored in a retrieval system or trans-
mitted in any form or by any means, electronic, mechanical, photocopying, recording,
scanning or otherwise, except as permitted under Sections 107 or 108 of the 1976 United
States Copyright Act, without the prior written permission of the Publisher. Requests to
the Publisher for permission should be addressed to the Permissions Department, Rockridge Press, 6005 Shellmound Street, Suite 175, Emeryville, CA 94608.

Limit of Liability/Disclaimer of Warranty: The Publisher and the author make no repre-
sentations or warranties with respect to the accuracy or completeness of the contents
of this work and specifically disclaim all warranties, including without limitation warranties of fitness for a particular purpose. No warranty may be created or extended by
sales or promotional materials. The advice and strategies contained herein may not be
suitable for every situation. This work is sold with the understanding that the Publisher
is not engaged in rendering medical, legal, or other professional advice or services. If
professional assistance is required, the services of a competent professional person
should be sought. Neither the Publisher nor the author shall be liable for damages
arising herefrom. The fact that an individual, organization or website is referred to in
this work as a citation and/or potential source of further information does not mean
that the author or the Publisher endorses the information the individual, organization
or website may provide or recommendations they/it may make. Further, readers should
be aware that Internet websites listed in this work may have changed or disappeared
between when this work was written and when it is read.

For general information on our other products and services or to obtain technical support, please contact our Customer Care Department within the U.S. at (866) 744-2665,
or outside the U.S. at (510) 253-0500.

Rockridge Press publishes its books in a variety of electronic and print formats. Some
content that appears in print may not be available in electronic books, and vice versa.

TRADEMARKS: Rockridge Press and the Rockridge Press logo are trademarks or registered
trademarks of Callisto Media Inc. and/or its affiliates, in the United States and other
countries, and may not be used without written permission. All other trademarks are the
property of their respective owners. Rockridge Press is not associated with any product
or vendor mentioned in this book.

INTERIOR AND COVER DESIGNER: Tina Besa
PHOTO ART DIRECTOR/ART MANAGER: Sue Bischofberger
EDITOR: Ada Fung
PRODUCTION EDITOR: Chris Gage
ILLUSTRATIONS: Chelsea Larsson

ISBN: Print 978-1-64611-071-1 | eBook 978-1-64611-070-4

R0

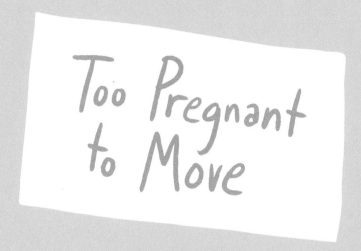

A PREGNANCY JOURNAL

BY CONZ PRETI

Illustrations by Chelsea Larsson

ROCKRIDGE
PRESS

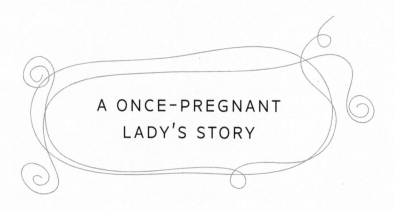

A ONCE-PREGNANT LADY'S STORY

Welcome to one of the most exciting, terrifying, confusing, and nauseating (quite literally) times of your life. The journey you're on is impossible to compare to any experience you've ever had before. Your body is actually growing a tiny human (or humans!), and every day, you will be in awe of what your amazing body and spirit are capable of doing. Next Tuesday will be just another day for everyone else around you, but for you, it might mean that you're helping little ears grow, or that a little set of eyes is developing inside your belly. How nutty is that?!

I still vividly remember how I felt when I saw those two pink lines for the first time. My initial reaction was sheer disbelief, so I took about 317 more pregnancy tests to make sure that I was, in fact, pregnant (spoiler alert: I was). Immediately after, I was in shock. Could I actually do this? Shock was quickly replaced by joy so intense that it had me in tears from laughing so much. That's how much of a roller-coaster ride pregnancy really is, and we're not just talking the first few days—it lasts (hopefully) for a full nine months.

I wish I had journaled during my first pregnancy. I would have loved to have a place to channel my raw and real emotions, and write down all the funny, weird, and incredible things that happened during my pregnancy. How amazing would it be to now have a record of my pregnancy so I could go back to reminisce on this time that was both so bewildering and so magical?!

In this journal, you will find plenty of space for you to record what's on your mind and how you're feeling throughout your pregnancy—and into the "fourth trimester," after you have your baby. There are pages for you to paste mementos like your sonograms and bump selfies (and maybe also a pregnancy test? I won't judge you for keeping it). At the end of each trimester, there are some additional blank pages so you can jot down your to-do list and questions for your doctor and friends—pregnancy brain is real, trust me! You'll find bits of advice and information on what to expect each trimester sprinkled throughout this journal, and a ton of reminders from me and other mamas who have been through this crazy ride that, even if you may feel unprepared or overwhelmed, you've got this!

Journaling will help give you perspective on how you're doing at each pregnancy milestone and will help illustrate how far you've come in the end. It will be something you'll want to keep forever and maybe even share with your children once they're old enough. Also, in this age where everything we see seems so Instagram perfect, it's good to have a place to vent about the low points of your journey, in addition to celebrating the highs.

So have fun. Make this journal your own. Scribble, draw, write all over it, use different colored pens, stickers, the whole thing. Or keep it all in black Sharpie—up to you! But whatever you do, keep it real and honest—use it as your place to decompress and relax, to laugh and cry. You're awesome, and you can do this!

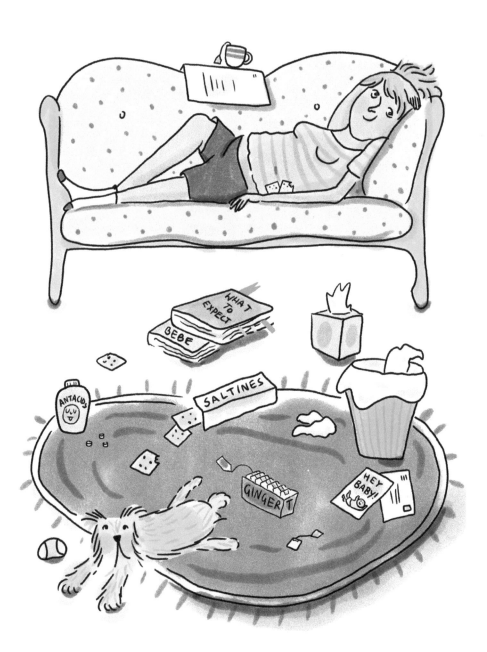

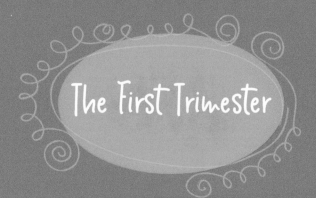

The First Trimester

WELCOME TO THE ROLLER COASTER OF PREGNANCY

WHAT YOU NEED TO KNOW ABOUT THE FIRST TRIMESTER

OMG! Congratulations! You're probably still rubbing your eyes in disbelief and trying to make sure that test really is positive. You're pregnant! Let's celebrate! What's that? You need to run to the bathroom to throw up? No worries, I'll wait.

Maybe you're feeling super excited and just want to fast-forward several months to when you'll have your adorable baby snuggled in your arms. Maybe you're feeling a little anxious about the unknown that is pregnancy, and your mind and heart are racing. There's no right or wrong way to feel. Take a deep breath and try to relax. Pregnancy is a special time, so try to just take it in and savor the next few months as much as you can.

If you ask me, this is the hardest trimester of the three. Somehow this one feels never-ending, compared with the other two. Add in all the rapid hormonal changes your body is going through, and this trimester could be pretty tough. This is when morning sickness is at its peak (they should really have called it around-the-clock sickness, amirite?!). You'll be super exhausted and wanting to take aaaalll the naps—which, if you work full-time, might be hard to explain to your boss. It's also when you'll have to kick some of your vices—sorry, no drinking or smoking allowed—and start eating healthier to nourish your lil' bean.

What to expect in the first couple of weeks will vary from person to person. Some people experience A LOT of symptoms early on, and some lucky ones breeze by without ever gagging once (so unfair!). Try not to drive yourself crazy by googling too much. What to expect on your first doctor's visit can also vary. Most doctors will do a blood test to check your HCG levels, aka the pregnancy hormone. You'll get a dating ultrasound as well, to see how many little babies you have in there and how far along you are. And get ready to become real comfortable with needles, because there will be a lot of poking and prodding for the next few months (sorry!).

Another thing you'll need to get used to is spending a lot of time in the bathroom, because one of the first symptoms is peeing a lot. A LOT. Like, waking up in the middle of the night multiple times to pee. Once, I dreamed I was about to sit on the toilet and woke up mere seconds away from actually wetting the bed. (I told you there was no such thing as TMI here.)

Uh, and is that the baby showing already?! Sorry, that's just bloat. Pregnancy slows down your digestion, so you'll be bloated and burpy. Sexy, huh? One way to combat this is to eat little meals throughout the day, so keep all the snacks nearby, but especially the saltines—they are going to be your BFF in these first few queasy weeks. Ask those around you to give you a little extra pampering. You deserve it—you *are* growing a human after all.

Eventually you will have a baby bump, so if you know you want to take bump photos, around Week 12 could be a good time to start. If you plan on wearing the same outfit for each photo, make sure you choose one that can accommodate a growing bump! No one wants a photo of themselves looking super uncomfortable in a too-tight shirt in Week 38.

Remember, no pregnancy is the same—so don't compare yourself to your friend, your neighbor, or even yourself in your previous pregnancy. Just enjoy the ride!

When and why did you decide to take a pregnancy test?
Where did you take it?

It is the most powerful creation for you to be able to have life growing inside of you. There is no bigger gift, nothing more empowering.

— BEYONCÉ,
musician and entrepreneur

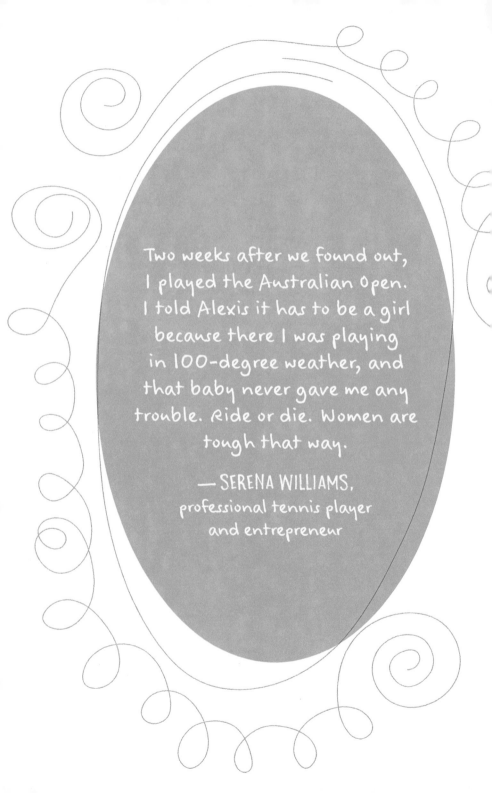

Two weeks after we found out, I played the Australian Open. I told Alexis it has to be a girl because there I was playing in 100-degree weather, and that baby never gave me any trouble. Ride or die. Women are tough that way.

— SERENA WILLIAMS,
professional tennis player
and entrepreneur

*Who was the first person you told? How did you feel when
you shared the news? What was their reaction?*

What kind of prep have you been doing since you found out? Are you reading any pregnancy books? Have you chosen an app to track your baby's development? Did you go with the fruits and veggies, weird animals, or some other strange weekly baby-size comparison?

The most annoying part of pregnancy is the fruit and veg shit: "Your baby is 6 inches. A pineapple!" What the fuck grocery store we at?

— CHRISSY TEIGEN,
model, author, and entrepreneur

FIRST SONOGRAM
(OR WHICH SPECK IS MY BABY?)

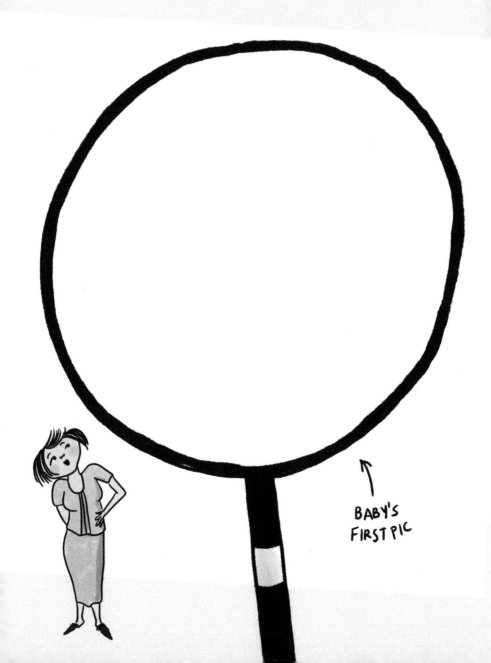

When I first heard my baby's heartbeat, I felt:

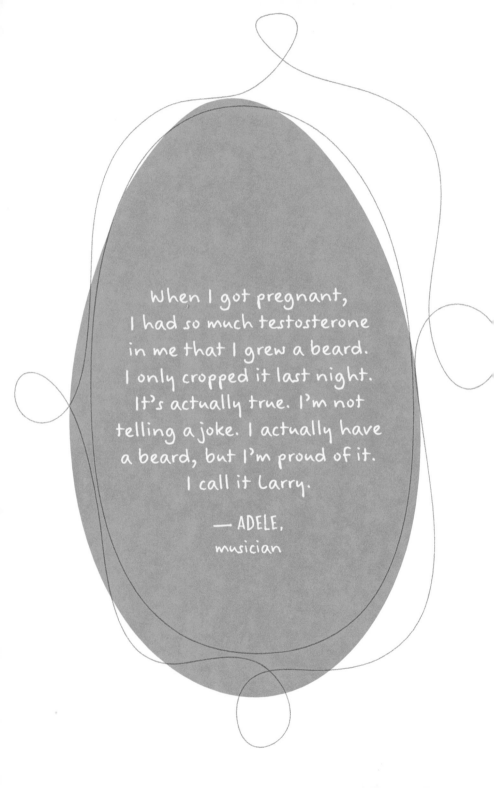

When I got pregnant,
I had so much testosterone
in me that I grew a beard.
I only cropped it last night.
It's actually true. I'm not
telling a joke. I actually have
a beard, but I'm proud of it.
I call it Larry.

— ADELE,
musician

Your baby is officially a fetus and not an embryo anymore. Hurray! What physical symptoms have you experienced this week? They peak now, so hang in there. It all gets better soon.

How are you feeling emotionally? What are some feelings you have that you didn't expect, and what feelings did you think you'd have but don't? Feel free to let the good and the bad out.

Stop saying, "We're pregnant." You're not pregnant! Do you have to squeeze a watermelon-sized person out of your lady-hole? No. Are you crying alone in your car listening to a stupid Bette Midler song? No.

— MILA KUNIS, actress

Thinking about names? Write down some of your faves here. You could have your partner write down theirs as well and see if any overlap! (Quick, while you still have time to convince them not to name the baby after their great-great-great-grandfather.)

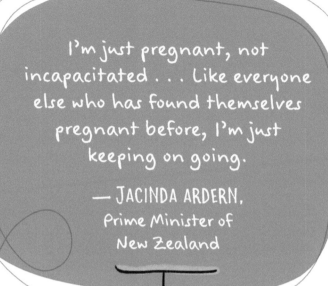
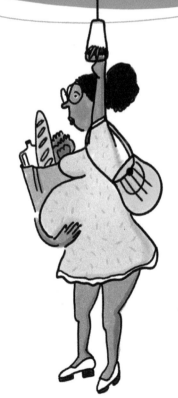

10 WAYS TO HIDE YOU'RE PREGNANT

1   If anyone asks why you're not drinking, say you're trying a dry month to get healthier. No one is going to question that.

2   Talk to the bartender ahead of time and let them know what's up. Have them serve you seltzer with lime and you can pretend to be drinking vodka soda all night.

3   Go into hiding. I'm serious! Avoiding situations where you would have to come clean is the best way to avoid having to do so. (This is ideal for all you introverts—now's the time to revel in your true self.)

4   Recruit your BFF. They can sneakily have your drink for you, or publicly commiserate about the food poisoning you both got from last night's street food to cover up the fact that you're running to the bathroom to puke all night.

5   Wear loose clothes to cover up the bloat. Do as actors do on TV and carry a large purse to disguise your tummy. Or try the ol' hairband trick so you can keep wearing your favorite pants. I'll let you google that one!

6   Keep snacks near you at all times to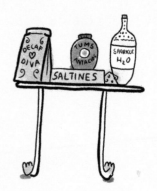
    avoid nausea and vomiting—telltale
    signs for busybodies to ask you if
    you're preggo. If you don't want to
    be obvious with a sleeve of saltines,
    try pretzels or sour candy. Seltzer is
    also a great friend right now.

7   Loudly tell everyone about what you did do on your
    awesome night out. No one needs to know that you didn't
    drink or eat sushi! Focus on the fun you're having and not
    what you're missing out on.

8   If someone asks why you're not having 18 cups of coffee
    like you used to, tell them you're using whitening stripes
    on your teeth and coffee is a no-no.

9   If worse comes to worst, fake a call and walk out of the
    situation. It works in the movies.

10 Write your own here:

    ....

    ....

    ....

    ....

How many naps have you taken this week? And how many naps do you wish you had taken?

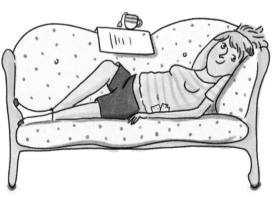

Pregnancy. It's just like a constant hangover.

— ELLIE KEMPER, actress

This is the last week of your first trimester! Have you announced yet? How did people react? If not, when and how do you plan on telling people?

People always say that pregnant women have a glow. And I say it's because you're sweating to death. I think they just tell pregnant women they're glowing to make them feel good about themselves.

— JESSICA SIMPSON,
musician and fashion designer

I HAVE SO MANY QUESTIONS

FIRST TRIMESTER THOUGHTS, MUSINGS, AND RANDOM TO-DOS

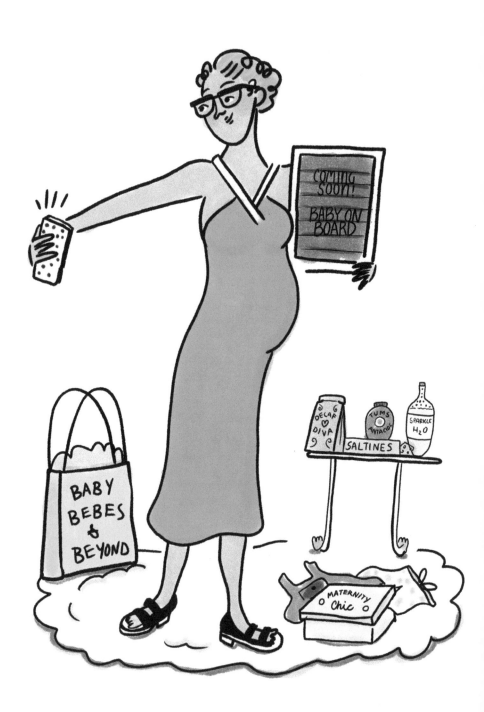

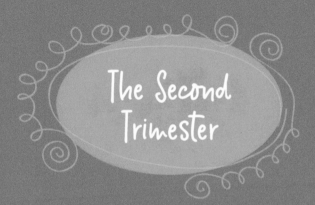

The Second Trimester

THAT PREGNANCY GLOW-UP

WHAT YOU NEED TO KNOW ABOUT THE SECOND TRIMESTER

Ah, the second trimester, or as I like to call it, the best trimester. The exhaustion and nausea from the first trimester slow down a bit, and you're not yet super huge and uncomfortable like you will be in the third trimester. Welcome to feeling more like yourself again!

By this point you may be comfortable sharing your news, finding out your baby's sex, and starting to really think about names and what your baby will be like. Your belly will become more of a noticeable bump—literally, it'll seemingly "pop" overnight. Strangers will be smiling at you left and right. They might even try to touch your bump; feel free to tell them no if that's not your thing. (Honestly, it's kinda weird, if you ask me.)

That bump of yours is only going to keep growing (and your boobs, and your . . . well, everywhere), so get yourself some comfy bras and clothes. Think stretchy fabrics and elastic waistbands!

As your baby grows, you'll have the quickening to look forward to, and I'm not talking about your reflexes. This is when you'll feel your little one move for the first time, which feels like little bubbles in your belly. When it starts will vary from person to person; if this isn't your first pregnancy, you'll feel baby move a lot sooner than you did the first time around.

The two big tests you need to look out for and mark on your calendar are the anatomy scan and the glucose test. Around Weeks 16 to 20 you'll have the anatomy scan, an ultrasound that evaluates and measures the baby's body parts, and to look at the positioning of your placenta. Assuming you haven't already done a blood test, you can also find out your baby's sex. If you don't want to find out, just make sure you tell the nurse to keep the sex a secret. Lean back, relax, and enjoy watching your little one moving around and posing for the camera (or the ultrasound wand—you get it!).

Between weeks 24 and 28 you'll take the glucose test, to test for gestational diabetes. You have to chug this super-concentrated sugary drink (ugh) and have your blood drawn and tested (double ugh, especially if you're like me and hate needles), so your doctor can measure your glucose levels and see how your body reacts to it. Take it easy on the cereal, muffins, and juice (or God forbid, donuts!) in the morning so you don't throw off your results and have to suffer through the more intensive three-hour-long test. Don't fast, just eat something healthy and protein-packed. If you do test positive, don't panic. Your doctor may want you to check your blood levels regularly and to see you more often during the last trimester just to make sure everything is A-okay. You may also have to tweak your diet and take medication to help your body. Make sure your doctor checks your sugar levels after birth as well.

If you're thinking of taking one, this is a great time to go on a babymoon, because soon you won't be able to (and won't want to) travel too far from home. Another thing to add to your to-do list is the baby registry and shower, if you decide you want one. If this is your second, third, fourth, or . . . (okay, you get it), you could have a baby "sprinkle" instead, just to get those basics that you may not have stashed away from your older kids.

This is a fun trimester, full of exciting milestones! Shout your news from the rooftops, give your cute ol' bump a congratulatory little self/group hug, and get ready for the adventures to come. But, you know, keep the antacids nearby because, TRUST ME, you'll still need them.

What nicknames do you have for your baby?

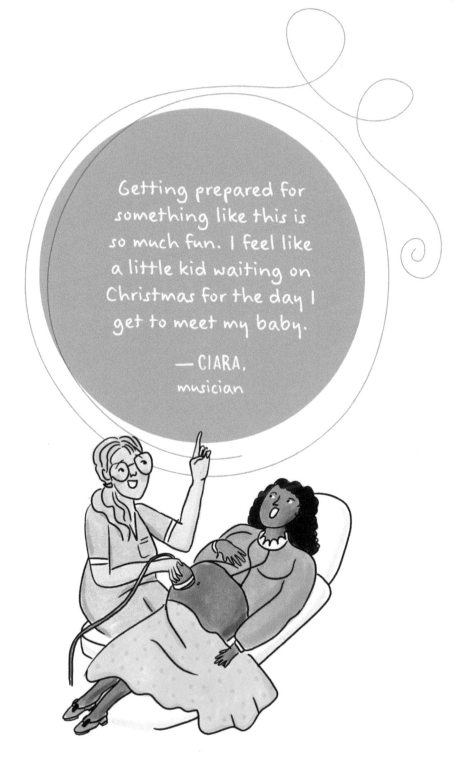

I had this thing for Entenmann's chocolate donuts. Somewhere during my pregnancy I gained something like nine pounds in two weeks and my doctor was like, "You know what it might be? Are you drinking a lot of juice?" I was like, "Yeah. That must be it." I was eating like a box a day of Entenmann's donuts.

—TINA FEY,
comedian and actress

What weird or super-specific food cravings have you had?

What steps have you taken to prepare for labor and child-birth? Have you maybe investigated the wide world of childbirth classes or looked into hiring a doula? (Or are you planning to just cross your fingers and push?)

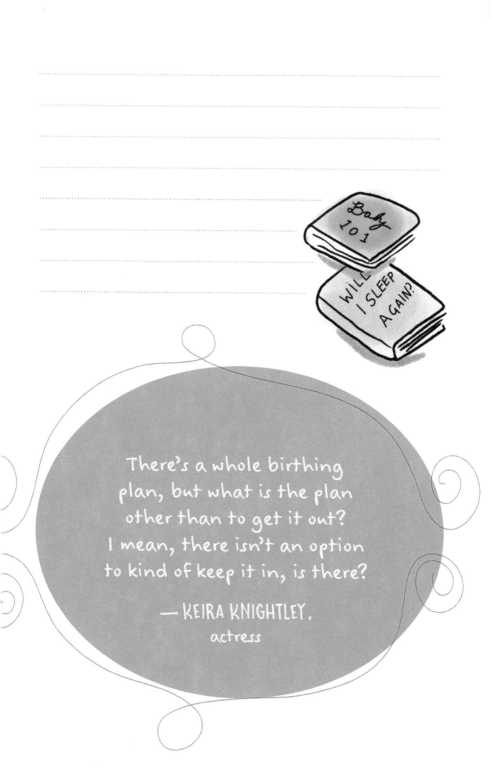

There's a whole birthing plan, but what is the plan other than to get it out? I mean, there isn't an option to kind of keep it in, is there?

— KEIRA KNIGHTLEY,
actress

What's a family tradition you're excited to share with your little one?

To describe my mother would be to write about a hurricane in its perfect power. Or the climbing, falling colors of a rainbow.

—MAYA ANGELOU, author

Have you felt your baby move? What emotions did it trigger in you?

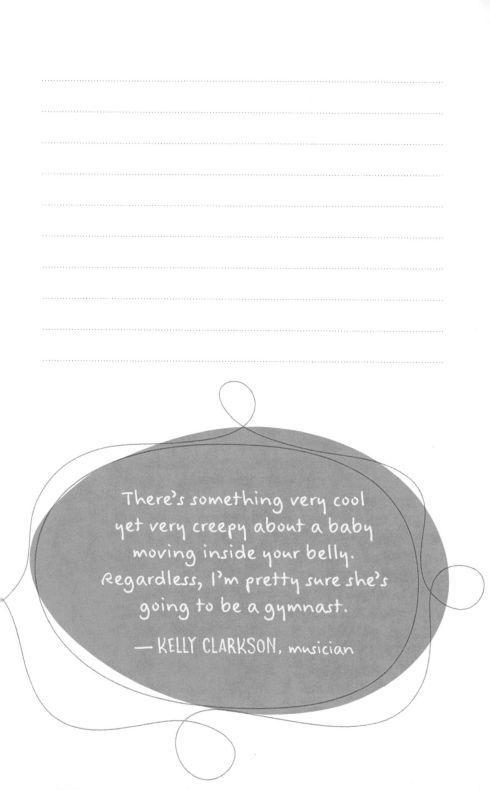

There's something very cool yet very creepy about a baby moving inside your belly. Regardless, I'm pretty sure she's going to be a gymnast.

— KELLY CLARKSON, musician

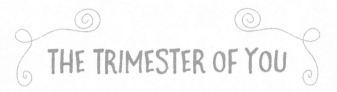

THE TRIMESTER OF YOU

This trimester is the BEST one because you finally get your energy back, but you aren't totally enormous yet—so, mama, it's time to enjoy it!

This is the time to nurture and take care of your growing body. Sign up for prenatal yoga or Pilates classes, or try some safe online classes you can do from the comfort of your own home. Trust me, your back is going to thank you in a couple of weeks.

Lather up and massage your belly with some cocoa butter to soothe any itchiness and prevent stretch marks. Sure, stretch marks are mainly genetic, so you might not really be able to avoid them, but it'll still feel really nice on your belly, plus it'll help you connect with your little one. Maybe you'll even feel some super-drastic movements—like a full-on belly ripple or a hand poking through, *Alien*-style.

Splurge on a nice prenatal massage. That hour or so you spend snoozing in a cozy room that smells like the lavender fields of Provence while someone rubs your sore muscles with warm oil is worth every penny. Or get a cute pedicure while you can still see your toes past your belly and splash out for the foot soak and massage. (Just make sure the salon is well-ventilated.) Treat yourself—you deserve it!

And hurray, your energy is back! That's your cue to go and have some fun. Go on, grab last-minute tickets to your favorite band's concert next week. Some doctors don't recommend super-loud shows when pregnant, but others say it's fine. (Can someone just invent noise-cancelling headphones for pregnant bellies?) If live music is not your thing, you can go to the movies, try a new restaurant (or revisit an old favorite), or host a game

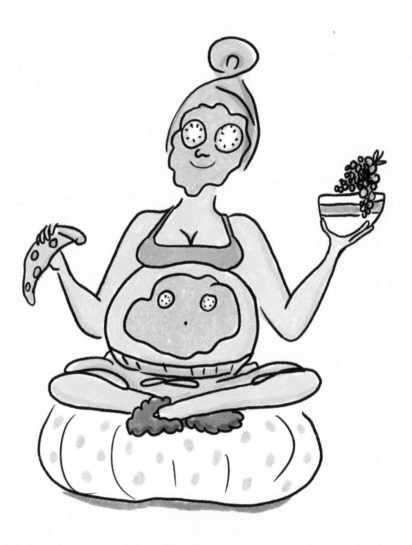

night—whatever your pleasure is. Put on your cutest maternity outfit, go out, and take advantage of strangers' kindness to snag the last table at your local hotspot!

Now's the time to do all of your favorite activities and plan new adventures. Hello, babymoon! Or babystaycation, whatever your speed. You're probably not gonna have the time or energy to do so after baby's here. You know, life with a newborn and all . . .

What fun activity or self-care thing do you want to do this week? Do you plan on taking a babymoon? Where to?

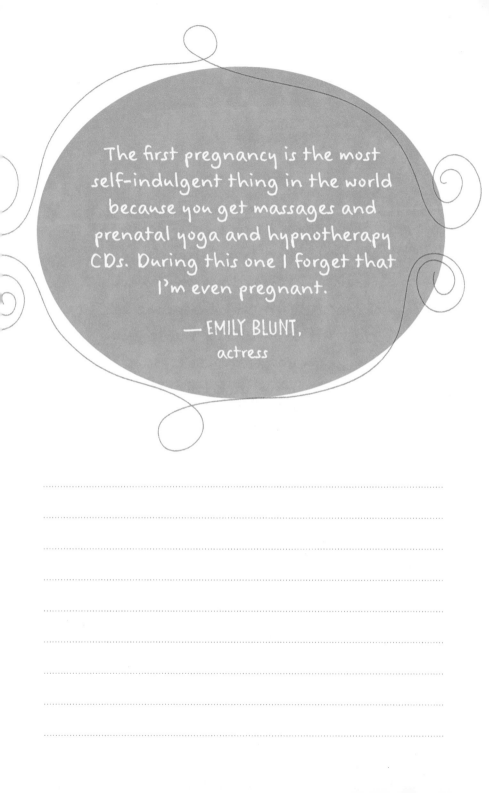

The first pregnancy is the most self-indulgent thing in the world because you get massages and prenatal yoga and hypnotherapy CDs. During this one I forget that I'm even pregnant.

— EMILY BLUNT,
actress

The baby hasn't even come out yet and I am already so resentful toward my husband. Especially when he asks me to do stuff around the house . . . "Hey, can you water the plants?" "I am not doing jack shit anymore; I'm busy making an eyeball!"

— ALI WONG,
comedian and actress

*Sing with me: "Whooooooaaa we're halfway theeeeeere!"
How are you feeling about the changes in your body? What
were you expecting and what caught you by surprise?*

SECOND SONOGRAM
(OR OMG, IT LOOKS LIKE A BABY!)

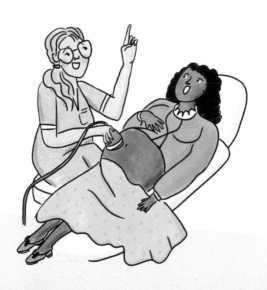

When I saw my baby on the ultrasound screen, I felt:

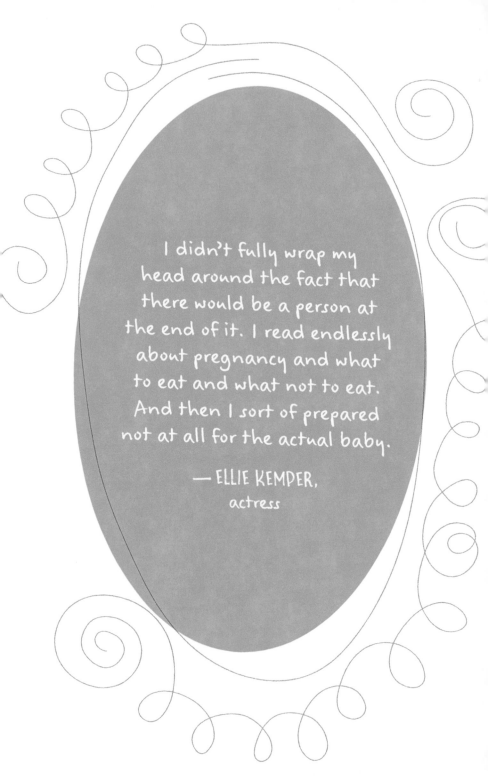

I didn't fully wrap my head around the fact that there would be a person at the end of it. I read endlessly about pregnancy and what to eat and what not to eat. And then I sort of prepared not at all for the actual baby.

— ELLIE KEMPER,
actress

Did you choose to find out your baby's sex? How did you feel when you found out? And if you're choosing to wait until birth, how are you explaining that choice to that one super-annoying relative who won't stop pestering you?

What's something you've found is the most different from the way movies and TV portray pregnancy? Besides, you know, everyone looking beautiful 24/7.

It's a joke if you think everybody's not hiding some secret shame about being anxiety-riddled or depressed at some point. We're all there, okay? Everybody's crazy. It's not a competition.

— KRISTEN BELL, actress

*Pregnancy dreams are **vivid** AF. What have been some weird ones you've had lately?*

I can smell electricity. I swear to
God I can smell the TV.

— AMANDA SEYFRIED,
actress

PREGNANCY AND BABY STUFF YOU NEED (AND WHAT YOU DON'T)

One of the most annoying things about being pregnant and having babies is the amount of stuff you need, or *think* you need, to survive this new part of your life. Some stuff people recommend *is* absolutely necessary (like diapers, for your baby and you), and some stuff they try to sell you is totally unnecessary and will just end up in the donate pile.

While pregnant, there's actually not that much you *absolutely* need. (You don't need a specialty pregnancy pillow—just construct one out of cushions and pillows you already have. Bonus, it'll be personalized to your own weird, achy body!) These are a few of my absolute must-haves:

» Maternity clothes are the one thing you should splurge on because you're growing a human and deserve to be as comfy as possible. Also, you'll probably be wearing your maternity pants well past birth because your uterus takes a while to shrink back, and you'll need the extra room for a pad the size of a small sofa (but more on that delight later!).
» Antacids, but do double-check with your doctor that you are cleared to take them. You cannot be too careful TBH.
» Prenatal vitamins that have DHA are key for your health and for your developing baby, so make sure you are taking yours daily! Take them on a full stomach—don't make the same mistake I did and take 'em on empty, ew.

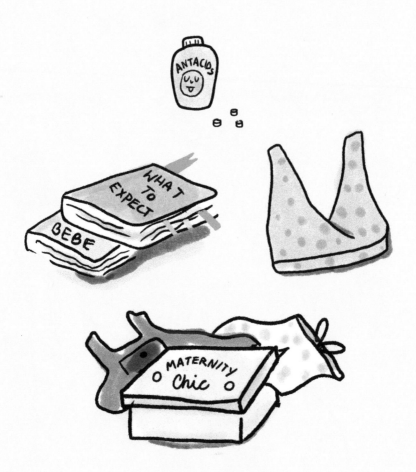

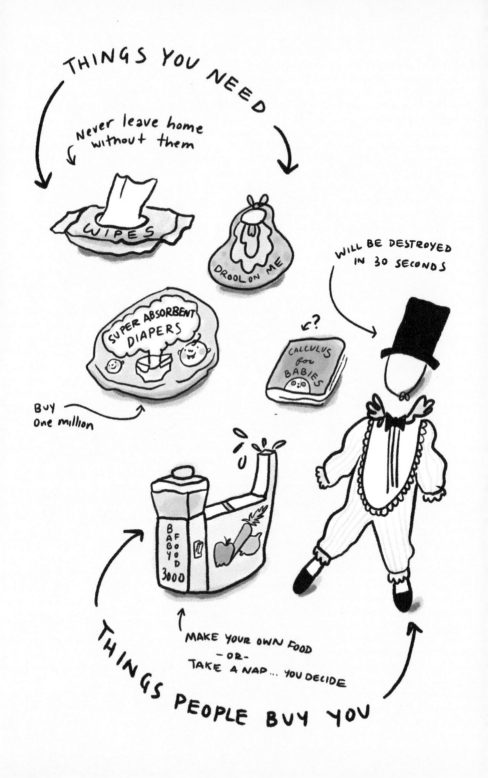

Newborns really don't need much. They definitely don't need a silver spoon or a hand-knitted Icelandic wool sweater (both totally real things that I got). Here's what you should get though:

» Diapers, butt cream, and wipes—A LOT of them because you have no idea how much pee and poop those little suckers expel out of their tiny bodies in the first couple of weeks.

» A thermometer—safety and health first!

» A safe sleeping place for all that snoozing; whether that's a fancy bassinet, a hand-me-down crib, a pack and play, or a co-sleeper, it's really up to you.

» Swaddles because newborns have a startle reflex that wakes them from sleep if they're not tightly wrapped like a burrito (or, ahem, take a few from the hospital).

» Something to carry them around in—be it a stroller, a baby carrier, or both.

» Some weather-appropriate clothes in a variety of sizes, though people will probably give you baby clothes whether you ask for them or not!

» A breast pump, just in case. You might already know what you want to do in terms of feeding, you might not (or your kiddo might have a different idea than you!). But it's good to have a pump handy and ready to use should you choose to breastfeed.

The rest you'll find out and buy as you go. Maybe your little one will be soothed by a pacifier or maybe they won't be into it. Maybe your kiddo will love chilling out in a swing or scream bloody murder if you put them in one. Too bad there's no way to ask it in advance! I get wanting to be as prepared as you can be, but try not to get sucked into buying a ton of things right off the bat. People love gifting things to new parents, so wait it out and buy as you need, or even better, look for hand-me-downs and used items, and don't forget to pay it forward.

I certainly spent a lot of time pregnant on camera. But I did have a job where no one cared. You can do your job massively pregnant if you choose to go down that road. It's fine. It'll be hilarious. It'll add to your comedy in ways that you never expected. Like when your elbows grow hair for no reason.

— SAMANTHA BEE,
comedian and
political commentator

Write down the things you plan on putting on your registry—and don't forget diapers! They're not glamorous, but you'll be glad to have a stash of them waiting for you when baby comes.

How many times did you pee today? (I promise that if you keep count, your mind will be blown.)

....

....

....

....

....

....

....

....

....

....

....

....

....

....

....

....

....

....

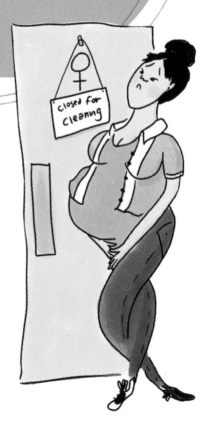

You are never alone when you are pregnant. I relish these moments when I feel my baby girl kick, until she's tap dancing on my bladder making me pee on myself.

— MOLLY SIMS, actress

What's the one value you most want to pass on to your little one?

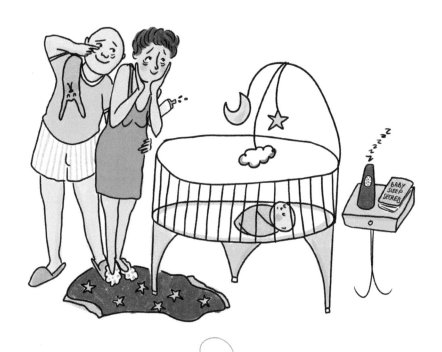

[My mother] had handed down respect for the possibilities—and the will to grasp them.

— ALICE WALKER, author

I HAVE SO MANY QUESTIONS

SECOND TRIMESTER THOUGHTS, MUSINGS, AND RANDOM TO-DOS

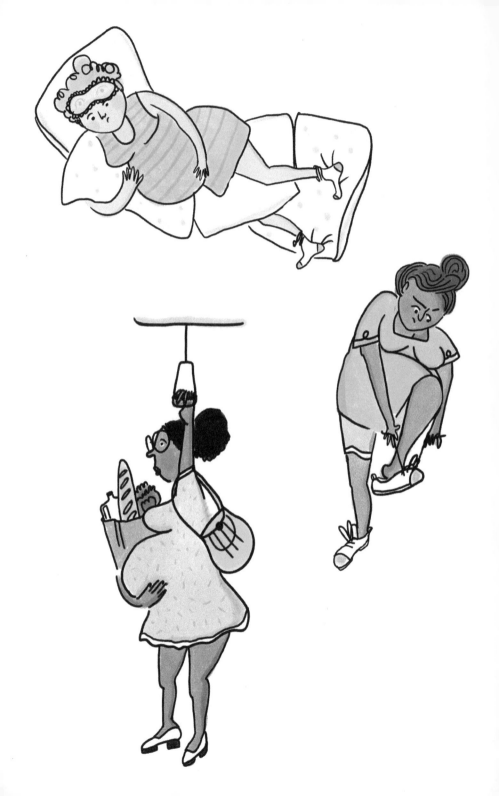

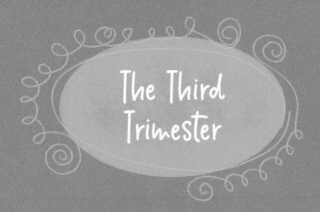

The Third Trimester

THIS JUST GOT REAL

WHAT YOU NEED TO KNOW ABOUT THE THIRD TRIMESTER

Sing with me: "It's the fiiiiinal countdown."

You've made it, mama. You are in your third trimester! Sooner than you know, you'll have your little one in your arms and you'll be staring down in disbelief at your baby and wondering just how on earth your body was able to create such a beautiful human. But before we get totally ahead of ourselves, let's talk about the final weeks and what to expect.

First of all, due dates are cute, but don't get too hung up on them. Your baby might plan on popping into the party early, or they might be fashionably late. If you go past yours (which is pretty common TBH), try not to be super bummed.

Remember when you were taking bump photos back in the second trimester thinking there was *no* way you could get any bigger? Hah! Sorry to be the bearer of bad news, but your belly might get so big that you'll become an expert in the pregnant-lady waddle. You'll basically be walking like a penguin, trying to not topple over. It's not cute. (Have I said I was sorry yet? I'm sorry.)

And, dear lord, the itching. As the skin around your belly stretches to accommodate your growing baby, you're going to get pretty itchy. Waddle over to Costco for a monster-size tub of cocoa butter, stat.

Around Weeks 35 to 37, your medical provider will test you for Group B Strep by swabbing both your vagina and anus (with different swabs!) to check for the bacteria. It sounds worse than it actually is. It takes seconds and I promise you'll barely notice what's happening. If you do test positive, which is totally normal, you'll need to have a shot administered before you deliver vaginally. So make sure you know what your results are in case you go into labor superfast and end up not seeing your regular medical team.

Around that same time your baby will turn head down and prepare to "drop"—aka descend into the birth canal. Are you psyched to have basically a bowling ball sitting right on top of your bladder and pelvis? Silver lining: You'll have more room in your ribcage to, y'know, breathe. If your baby is stubborn (like mine was), they might decide to stay head-up, in what's known as the breech position. You'll want to keep constant tabs on baby's position because there are risks with going into labor with a baby in breech. To help, you can try acupuncture, do some Spinning Babies exercises, or opt for an ECV, which is when they manually turn your baby from outside your belly. Scheduling a C-section for peace of mind is also an option. Know that babies can turn at any point, even during labor.

By now you should have your birth plan printed out, know the best route to your hospital or birthing center, have a pediatrician picked out, and have the car seat installed. Yeah, this trimester is a lot about planning and organizing, which maybe isn't your idea of a fun way to spend the last few weeks before you become a mom. But when you go into labor, you won't be thinking straight and your partner will be too busy trying to make you comfortable (more backrubs!), so have as much ready ahead of time to reduce the panic and running around in circles during those overwhelming hours (or minutes) before you leave the house.

Are you ready? Let's have a baby!

When do you think baby will come? How about your partner? Family and friends? Write down everyone's guesses and send a little present to the person who gets the closest.

....

....

....

....

....

....

....

....

....

....

....

....

....

....

....

....

....

No one's really doing it perfectly. I just think you love your kids with your whole heart, and you do the best you possibly can.

— REESE WITHERSPOON,
actress and producer

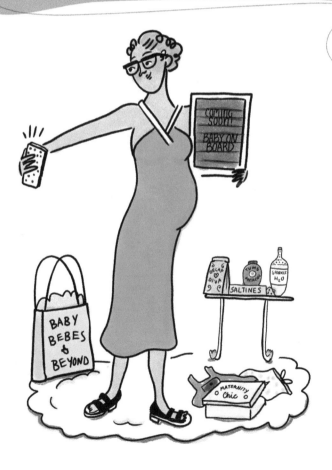

Is your baby all up in your ribs? Space is getting tight in there! Where else does it feel like baby is jamming up on? List your various discomforts and complaints here so you can guilt trip your kiddo later.

"Does this baby make
me look fat?"

— AMY SCHUMER,
comedian and actress

One thing that happens when you're pregnant is that as your stomach starts to stretch, it itches! So I have to keep my belly really lubricated. Every morning, there's a buttering ceremony after I get out of the shower. It's really like basting a turkey with body butter.

—PADMA LAKSHMI, author and television host

Have you had any randos come up to touch your baby bump or ask really intrusive questions about your pregnancy? What did you say to them? (And what do you really wish you had said to their face?)

....

....

....

....

....

....

....

....

....

....

....

....

....

....

....

....

....

....

CREATING A BIRTH PLAN

Everyone has different preferences about things, so why would a birth plan be any different? Whatever your mother or sister wanted or did likely won't be the same as what you want, and you shouldn't feel pressured to do things a certain way just because they did. I love the Amy Poehler motto "Good for her! Not for me." Just repeat that to yourself, over and over, if you find yourself trapped in a conversation with a well-meaning friend about what you should or shouldn't do during childbirth (or, you know, feel free to politely say it out loud).

It's your birth, it's your experience, so take some time to think about what you want that day. Some know they want no pain meds at all; others know that they're going to want that epidural ASAP. Some will create a playlist ahead of time, and some download TV shows to watch on their tablets, while others won't even think to plan ahead for entertainment. Some will want a vaginal birth; others know they will have to schedule a C-section for health reasons. Some might choose birth at home; some at a hospital. (And a select few may think they have a plan, but end up having their babies in the back of a car, in an apartment building lobby . . .)

My only advice is for you to be ready for any type of birth and to be prepared to be flexible. So even though you want a vaginal birth with no painkillers, make sure you read a little bit about what happens during a C-section *juuust* in case you need one. Knowledge is power, and it's especially true when it comes to birthing babies. The more knowledge you have, the better you'll be able to advocate for yourself, stay calm through labor, and recover from the hard work your body will go through.

Have you thought about your birth plan? Do you want meds or nothing? Do you have a playlist ready or do you want total silence? Write down your thoughts here.

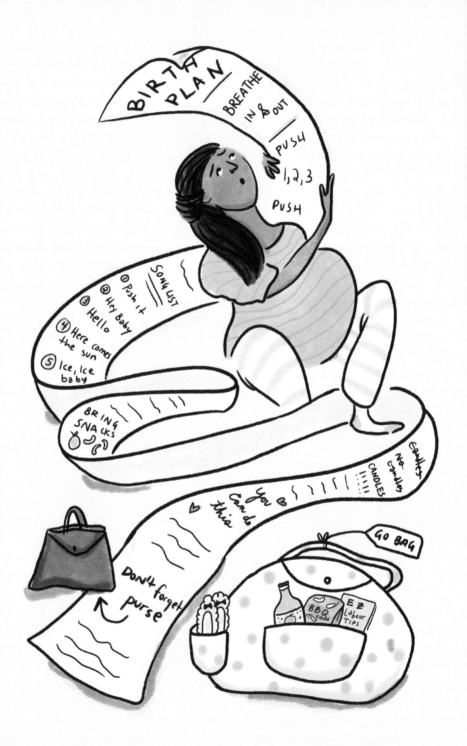

Have you tried playing music for your little bean? What are some of their favorite genres or artists?

....

....

....

....

....

....

....

....

[Motherhood is] the biggest gamble in the world. It is the glorious life force. It's huge and scary— it's an act of infinite optimism.

— GILDA RADNER,
comedian and actress

MY AWESOME PREGNANT SELFIE

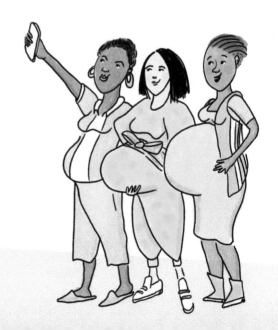

This is when I felt the most beautiful/powerful/awesome during pregnancy:

....

....

....

....

....

....

....

....

....

....

....

....

....

....

....

....

....

....

You might be getting Braxton-Hicks by now, aka practice contractions. Jot down how they feel so you can compare them to the contractions you get closer to your due date— it'll help you figure out if they're the real deal. (Oh, and tell your doc, obviously!)

I felt like when I was having contractions, I envisioned my child pushing through a very heavy door. I imagined this tiny infant doing all the work, so I couldn't think about my own pain. We were talking. I know it sounds crazy, but I felt a communication.

— BEYONCÉ,
musician and entrepreneur

What do you hope your baby will get from you and your partner—both in terms of looks and personality? And what do you hope they'll skip?

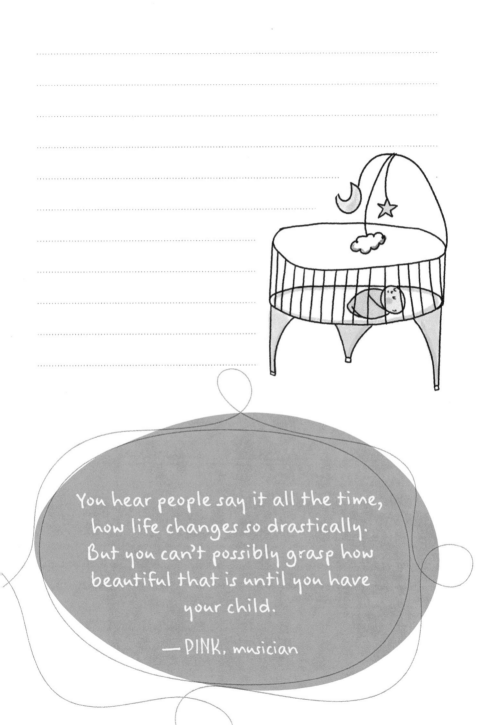

You hear people say it all the time, how life changes so drastically. But you can't possibly grasp how beautiful that is until you have your child.

— PINK, musician

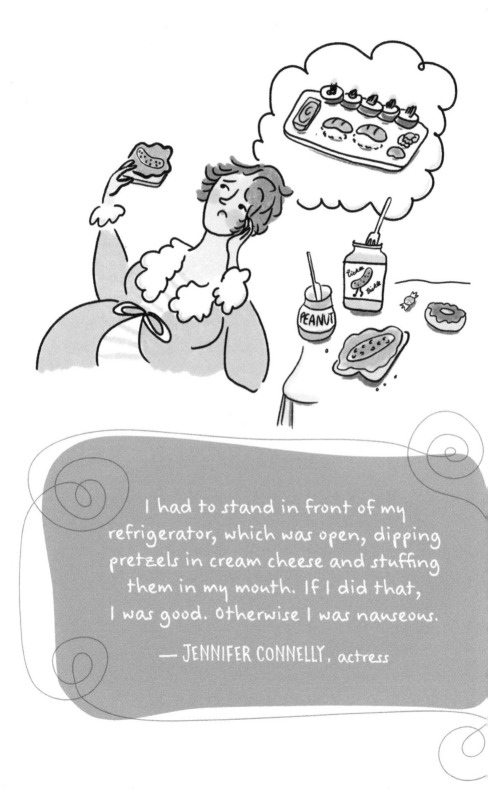

I had to stand in front of my refrigerator, which was open, dipping pretzels in cream cheese and stuffing them in my mouth. If I did that, I was good. Otherwise I was nauseous.

— JENNIFER CONNELLY, actress

What have you been doing in the middle of the night when insomnia hits? Trying any new recipes? Staying up going through your to-do list? Or just enjoying feeling your baby move?

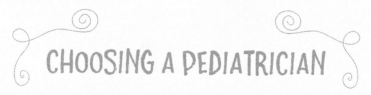

CHOOSING A PEDIATRICIAN

By now you are probably BFFs with your gyno because you've been seeing them so often. However, you're going to need a new medical BFF on speed dial soon—a doctor for your little one. You'll need to take your kiddo to their new doctor within the first few days of giving birth, so now's the time to look for a pediatrician. How to choose one? I go by three rules:

» Distance to where you live: Right after having a baby, you won't want to (or maybe won't even be able to) drive an hour and back with a newborn. So try to pick someone who is nearby. You'll also be thankful when your kiddo is sick and you need to be seen ASAP.

» Word of mouth: If you have family or friends nearby who have kids, ask them who their pediatrician is. If you have no one around, you can ask a local mom group on Facebook—they are always a good resource. Or ask your OBGYN—they know *all* the good pediatricians in town!

» Internet reviews: This is the last thing you should check, because, y'know, the Internet can be kinda iffy. But you'll be glad you found out that doctor so-and-so has a three-hour wait time, because no one has time for that.

Your child's doctor should be someone who makes you feel comfortable, and whose advice and recommendations you trust. Also, they should be someone who takes the time to answer all your new-mom questions—and, oh boy, you'll have them. So don't feel like you're going overboard if you want to interview a bunch of pediatricians before picking one.

What questions do you want to ask a prospective pediatrician? Write them down here so you don't forget.

*Have you peezed? You know . . . sneezed and peed a little.
It'll be our secret, but how many times have you peed
your pants this pregnancy? And where was the most
embarrassing place it happened?*

It's a great thing about being pregnant—you don't need excuses to pee or to eat.

— ANGELINA JOLIE, actress and filmmaker

Breathe. Everything is about to change, and it's a beautiful thing. Gather support. In fact, gather all the support. You need postpartum support more than any baby item. Real talk. Gather your village.

— BRANDI SELLERS-JACKSON, doula

I'm sure you've gotten all kinds of baby advice, but what has been the weirdest or most random bit of advice someone has given you?

SUPER ABSORBENT DIAPERS

Buy
One million

What are you most looking forward to about giving birth?
And what are you most terrified of?

A lot of women tried to freak me out. They tried to freak me out about childbirth by saying, "Ali, did you know that you're gonna poop on the table?" . . . It makes sense, like, that you—that that happens because when you're in labor, you push, you push, you push, and your husband will be asked to assist in the labor by lifting up your leg, which subsequently turns into a soft-serve lever. You just shit on the floor in front of the love of your life.

— ALI WONG, comedian

How are you feeling right now? Jot down your physical pains and your emotions as your due date approaches.

Oh, my God, I'm crying at everything lately. I'm watching Extreme Makeover: Home Edition, and I was crying so hard. There's no shame in that. I'm crying at everything. The wind will blow a branch and I'm like, aw, nature.

— AMY POEHLER,
comedian and actress

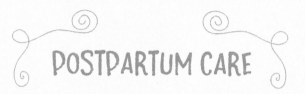

POSTPARTUM CARE

Let's get super real about what's about to go down, okay?

You're gonna have a baby, they are gonna be all squishy and adorable, and you won't believe you just did that. But you did, and your body will remind you. You'll be exhausted and hungry probably. Also, sore. And dealing with all the postpartum hormones. And the bleeding—yes, the postpartum bleeding. It's all quite a bit messy, huh?

If you're going to be giving birth at a hospital or birthing center, TAKE HOME AS MUCH AS YOU CAN! This is not a drill. And it's not rude! So many people told me this and I felt weird about it and then I realized that the nurses were basically expecting us to loot the room, forcing us to take more diapers for the baby, and enormous pads and mesh underwear for me. So take everything—the nose sucker for baby and the peri bottle for you.

Also, take advantage of the fact that you will have an arsenal of nurses who have a ton of knowledge on newborns, so ask them all your pressing questions. They can teach you how to swaddle your baby into a tight burrito, tell you how many poops and pees to look for in the first week, how to take care of your C-section incision, how to clean your vagina, and basically how to deal with everything you have either completely forgotten from birth class or never had any clue about, but that they've dealt with one million and one times.

Eat. Nourish your body. You just went through a marathon that ended with a sprint. (Not that I know anything about running, but I do know about birthing babies.) Your body needs extra TLC right now. Eat that burger with fries, or the sushi you've been craving for nine months. Go ahead and crack a bubbly and cheers with your partner. Celebrate with your favorite slice of chocolate cake. You did it!!!

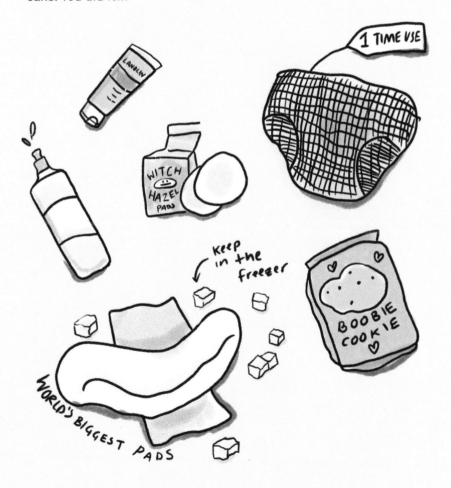

What things do you want to have on hand at home for your postpartum recovery? Make a list and then order someone to go get them for you. (What? You're far too exhausted to go anywhere now.)

No one told me I would be
coming home in diapers too.

— CHRISSY TEIGEN,
model, author and entrepreneur

What's been the most awesome thing about being pregnant? And what's been the worst?

So never compare yourself or your story to anyone else's. You are unique and your story makes you who you are today. Your fertility, pregnancy, birth story, and parenting styles are your decisions and experiences and no one else's.

— KIRI VASALES,
fashion designer

How many people have asked you if you've had the baby already? Who has been the most annoying? You can write down your make-believe hit-list here; we won't tell.

I gotta be honest it's really irritating to hear people say, "God, you've been pregnant forever" . . . I'm making a baby, not ramen noodles.

— AMBER ROSE, model

What creative things have you tried to get this effing baby out of you?

GO BAG

BBQ Chips

E Z Labour Tips

Giving birth is like taking your lower lip and forcing it over your head.

—CAROL BURNETT, comedian and actress

I HAVE SO MANY QUESTIONS

THIRD TRIMESTER THOUGHTS, MUSINGS, AND RANDOM TO-DOS

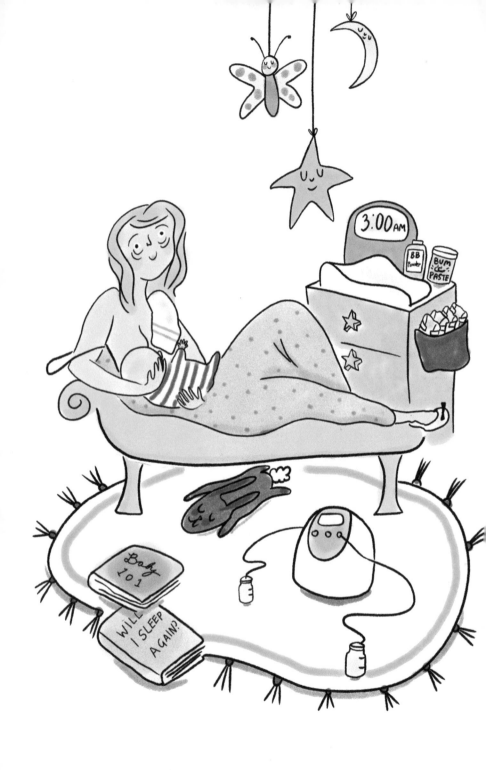

SLEEP? WHAT'S SLEEP?

WHAT YOU NEED TO KNOW ABOUT THE FOURTH TRIMESTER

You've birthed a baby, so give me a high five, mama! Now that baby is out, it's time to put the difficulties and discomfort of pregnancy behind you and just enjoy them and snuggle them, except . . . what's that? Oh, babies don't necessarily know they are in the outside world, and so this is *aaaalll* gonna be a huge adjustment for them (and you)? Yep. This is why newborns love to be swaddled tightly, fall asleep in the car (it's the motion), and are up all night. They wanna keep enjoying everything that made them feel warm and safe inside your comfy belly, just like they've been feeling for months. Can you blame them? That's why the first three months of new parenthood are called the fourth trimester (just when you thought you were done with those).

As for you, your body has gone through quite a journey, so try not to neglect your recovery, even in the whirlwind of caring for a newborn. Don't expect to get back in your skinny jeans immediately. You're carrying around a lot of water, plus your uterus needs to shrink down to its normal size and settle back under your pelvis. So be kind to yourself and appreciate everything you've done to grow all these fingers and toes.

It's going to be hard in a lot of ways. The sleep deprivation is really tough, and nothing really prepares you for it. Also, the hormonal fluctuations can wreak havoc on your emotions, so I encourage you . . . actually, no, I *urge* you to write and speak about everything you are feeling. It will help you get through your new-parent anxieties and also help those around you understand what you are dealing with.

Get all the help you can. Whether that comes in the shape of a loving grandma who has free time to give or hiring a professional baby nurse to give you a couple of extra hours of sleep, don't be afraid to ask for help. Know that it doesn't make you any less capable or a "bad mom" if you choose to have an extra set of hands in the house.

If you haven't thought about joining a postpartum mom group, now might be a good time to see if there are any around you. I know that you're feeling raw and vulnerable, so leaving the house might seem scary—add a cranky newborn to the mix, and you might feel like hibernating forever. But it's really good to get out, breathe some fresh air, and talk with people who are going through the same thing as you. Also, you *know* the other new moms won't give a crap about your spit-up stains or your leaky boobs. (Isn't motherhood sexy?)

Don't forget to enjoy this new time in your life. Yes, it's going to be chaotic, messy, and sometimes straight-up scary. But it's also wonderful, because that baby you are holding in your arms? You made that! All those days you wondered what they might look like, smell like, be like? They're in the past—you are a mom (or mommy, mama, mami, whatever you decide to go by), and you should embrace that.

These three months just fly by, and it'll all be a bit of a blur because you're so tired. But, deep breaths, you can do this, everything will be okay!

THE TEENIEST, MOST PERFECT NEWBORN FOOTPRINTS

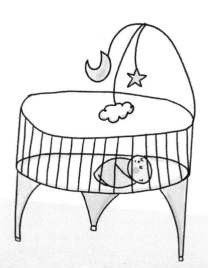

When I first held my baby, I felt:

What was labor and childbirth like? Write down your birth story here so you can share it with your little one when they're older.

I feel like, when I arrive at the hospital, I want a glass of whiskey, I want the epidural in my back, and I want to get hit in the face with a baseball bat.

—KRISTEN BELL, actress

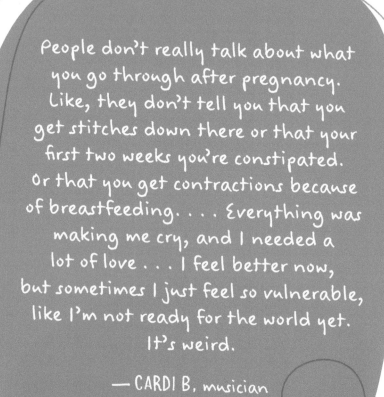

People don't really talk about what you go through after pregnancy. Like, they don't tell you that you get stitches down there or that your first two weeks you're constipated. Or that you get contractions because of breastfeeding. . . . Everything was making me cry, and I needed a lot of love . . . I feel better now, but sometimes I just feel so vulnerable, like I'm not ready for the world yet. It's weird.

— CARDI B, musician

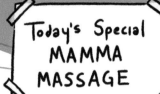

Today's Special
MAMMA
MASSAGE

How are you doing, mama? How are you dealing with the roller coaster of postpartum emotions? Remember to take a little time for self-care, even if it's just taking a longer shower than normal.

Where's baby's favorite place to nap?

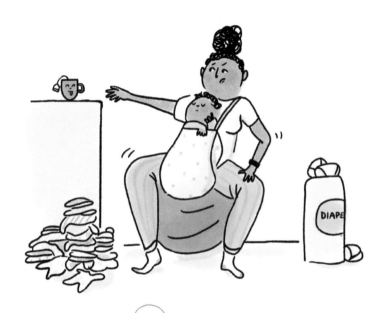

I realize this is the most obvious thing in the world to say, but sometimes it hits me all of a sudden that he won't be a baby forever. This simple fact breaks my heart every single time I think about it.

— VIOLET GAYNOR,
cofounder of The Glow

BREASTFEEDING IS FRIGGIN' HARD

You might have decided you don't even want to try breastfeeding, so if that's the case, you can feel free to skip this part. However, if you are giving it a go, or are dead set on doing only boobs, let me tell you something: Breastfeeding is friggin' hard.

Some babies are pros at it, some need a little guidance, and others are just straight up not into it. So just like you went into planning your birth with an open mind, I recommend going into your breastfeeding journey with the same openness and A LOT of extra clean shirts and burp cloths near you. You're gonna need them! Also, nipple cream—dear lord, do not forget to stock up on the nipple cream.

See a lactation consultant shortly after delivering. If you have your baby at a hospital, they might have one available to see you in your room. They are pros at teaching you how to properly latch your baby—spoiler alert: Babies are not born knowing how to nurse.

Lactation consultants are AWESOME. Seriously, consider keeping one on speed dial. They can show you different ways of holding your baby while you feed them, which will be great for your lower back and shoulders because you'll be doing a lot of sitting and holding, so a little change will go a long way. They can troubleshoot a variety of nursing issues you might be having. They can also help you find the right breast pump and flange size, once you're ready for that. But more than technical support, they can reassure you and cheer you on in the early weeks when you and baby are figuring out this whole new world of breastfeeding.

Breastfeeding can also be hard in unexpected ways. You might've thought that you'd be totally cool with plopping a boob out in public, but now that you're in your new postpartum body, you find yourself doing advanced contortionism to cover yourself. You might feel like a total badass feeding your child with your own body, or it might trigger anxiety because you can't tell if they're getting enough food. You'll definitely feel that sweet, sweet oxytocin running through your body as your baby sucks on your nip, but you also might feel annoyed that you can't really get away from baby for too long because newborns eat ALL THE TIME. So even though breastfeeding might be everything you ever wanted to do, it's okay to feel like it also kinda, well, sucks.

In a blink of an eye, they'll start getting bigger and heavier. Know that every adorable chubby roll on their body was all your doing! (Your partner and mom and whoever else is wise enough to feed you snacks while you nurse can have partial credit.)

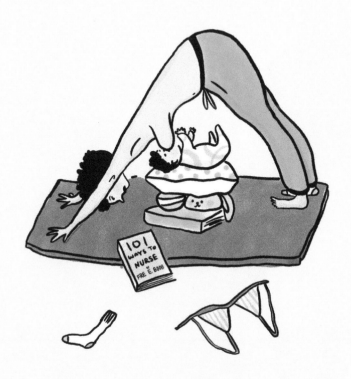

How are you feeling? Is the whole feeding, sleeping, changing thing feeling easier? (This is a safe space. Let it aallll out.)

Being a modern mom is confusing as fuck. In some ways, we are better equipped than our mothers. We have more in our tool belts, but it's a trick. I'm expected to do what my dad was doing and what my mom was doing, but I'm not sure who is making me do that except me. So, of course I feel like I'm doing a mediocre job at everything.

—GRETA LEE, actress

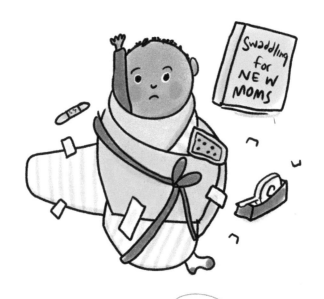

Baby brain is real.
I should not be permitted
to operate heavy equipment
including iPhones.

— OLIVIA WILDE,
actress and director

All right, what are some funny stories from your first month together? You know, like that time you caught poop in your hands?

....

....

....

....

....

....

....

....

....

....

....

....

....

....

....

....

....

....

What is the best advice you've gotten from other moms or experts that you want to make sure to pass along to others?

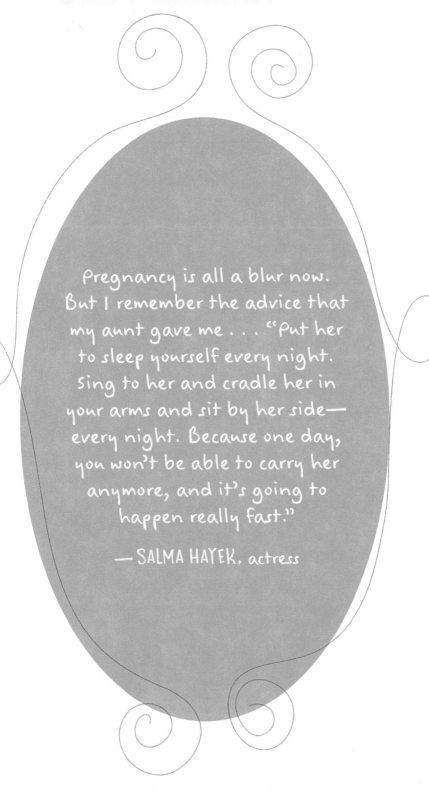

Pregnancy is all a blur now. But I remember the advice that my aunt gave me . . . "Put her to sleep yourself every night. Sing to her and cradle her in your arms and sit by her side—every night. Because one day, you won't be able to carry her anymore, and it's going to happen really fast."

—SALMA HAYEK, actress

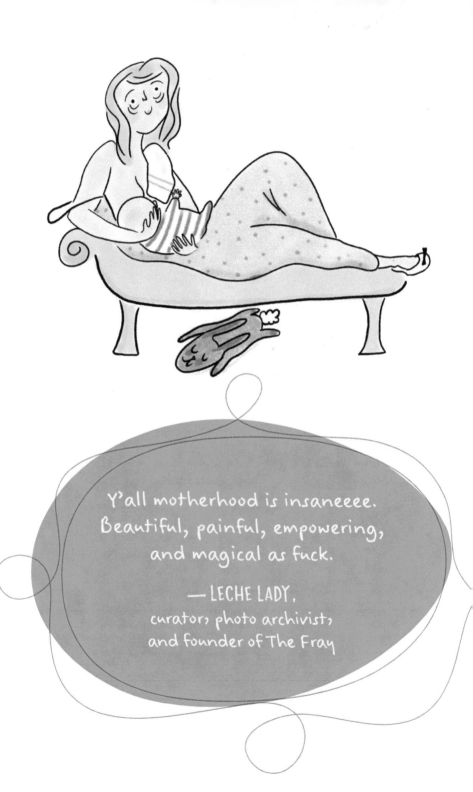

Are we tummy-timing? How does your baby react to being face down?

....

....

....

....

....

....

....

....

....

....

....

....

....

....

....

....

....

....

How does your baby react to being outside? Are they fascinated by the new views or are they total homebodies?

One of the most magical parts
of being a mom has been the rebirth
of my perception. As I watch Viva
experience things for the first time,
I find myself observing the world more
acutely with a reemerging sense of
awe and amusement.

— PIERA GELARDI,
cofounder of Refinery29

What do you call your baby? Sure, you gave them a lovely name, but I bet you they get called anything but that.

I swear, if I could eat my children, I would. I'd consume them like some beast in a Hieronymus Bosch painting, but in a friendlier, more mom-like way. Their little bodies make me salivate. It takes everything I have not to swallow them whole.

— AMY POEHLER, comedian and actress

....

....

....

....

....

....

....

....

How's baby sleeping? How are you sleeping?

Everything I've done for the
past five years, I've done
while sleep-deprived.

— GWEN STEFANI,
singer, actress, and producer

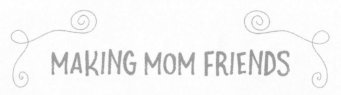

MAKING MOM FRIENDS

Making friends is hard. Making friends as an adult is almost impossible. So I get that you might think that making mom friends is basically like climbing Everest without shoes. I won't lie—it can be overwhelming and hard, especially because we all have different ways of parenting and make different choices when it comes to our kids.

Buuuuuuut, it's worth it. Having someone to message at 2 a.m. with a photo of your baby's poop, asking if it looks the same as their baby's, will be good for you and everyone around you. They'll be a great resource for tips, late-night vent sessions, product recommendations (maybe even some freebies!), and just over-all support.

And look, it doesn't have to be an IRL group of moms. It can be your due-date-month bumpers in the dark corner of the internet (aka Reddit), it can be a Facebook group of moms around your area, or it can be someone you met at your birthing class or hospital tour who you text only when you need to. You can make your own village any way that suits you.

If you choose to go the IRL route, make sure people are on the same page as you before making it a regular meet-up to avoid awkward moments. If vaccines are a big deal for you, speak up so everyone knows where you stand. Worse than making mom friends is having to break up with them.

Plus, once the babies are a little older and you can leave them with a caregiver without having a mini heart attack, you can go out with your new friends who will understand why you have a 9 p.m. curfew and your hair is all dry shampoo. (#nojudgment.)

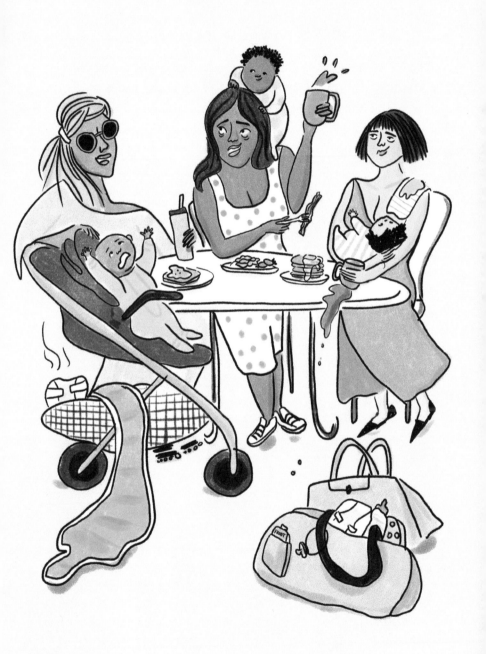

What's something a fellow parent-in-the-trenches told you or did for you that helped you feel more reassured?

....

....

....

....

....

....

....

....

....

....

....

....

....

....

....

Does your little one already have a favorite bedtime book? Or have you made up a bedtime song they love? Write down the lyrics before you forget!

There is something so magical about having a baby in the house. Time expands and contracts; each moment holds its own little eternity.

— MICHELLE OBAMA, Former First Lady

Your baby is not a newborn anymore! What were some of your favorite moments from these last few weeks?

I've learned that it's way harder
to be a baby. For instance,
I haven't thrown up since the '90s
and she's thrown up twice since we
started this interview.

— EVA MENDES, actress

I HAVE SO MANY QUESTIONS

FOURTH TRIMESTER THOUGHTS, MUSINGS, AND RANDOM TO-DOS

ACKNOWLEDGMENTS

A big shout-out to all the mom friends I've made along the way—you've kept me grounded and sane. Thank you to my parents for everything they've done—I get it now, I really do. To my husband, whom I couldn't have done any of this without—thank you for your patience, care, and love. And to our son, thank you for making me a mom. I never thought I wanted to be part of this crazy joy ride, but you show me every day that I was meant to share my life with you. I love you all forever.

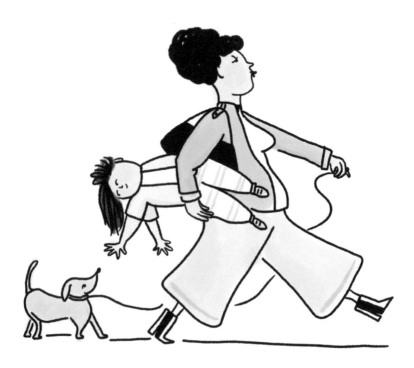

ABOUT THE AUTHOR

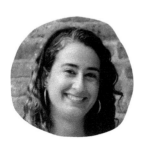

Conz Preti is a writer and a journalist from Argentina, currently living in New York City with her husband, son, and two pups. After a decade building international digital journalism teams, her decision to start a family led to a quandary: How do you raise a good person without messing up? The personal rewards of parenthood are expected. The challenges and their solutions post-delivery through adolescence are unique and unknown. As a mother, she has found joy in her family and the community of parents she now finds herself a member of. Together they are building modern childhood for their offspring in the big city.

ABOUT THE ILLUSTRATOR

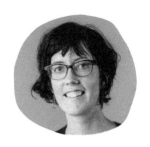

Chelsea Larsson is an illustrator by night, a ux writer by day, and a mom all the time. She lives in Berkeley, California, with her husband and two-year-old daughter. She's mostly got it together, except for when her daughter is hangry. Or when she is hangry. Basically, snacks are the only thing keeping her family intact. Her work has been in *Bravery* magazine and *Illustoria* magazine, and she's the creator of *Life Is Boobiful*, a zine about breastfeeding.

CPSIA information can be obtained
at www.ICGtesting.com
Printed in the USA
BVHW050306081219
565881BV00001B/1/P